NURSING HOME SECRETS

Nursing Home Secrets

REGINA WATKINS

Regina's Corner

Dear Reader, I do understand the frustrations of knowing that a family member may need to be placed in a long-term care facility, and once they are there, it continues to be an ongoing emotional process.

I experience the same feelings when my 95-year old grandmother and my great-aunt (my grandmother's sister) were placed in a skilled nursing facility; the only difference was my experience and comprehensive knowledge of care planning and knowing what questions to ask, allowed me the opportunity to speak on their behalf while overseeing their quality of care.

I have worked in nursing homes, memory care, and assisted living facilities for over twenty years. During this time, I was a part of a multidisciplinary team (MDT), which is a group of healthcare professionals who work together in planning the care of residents. The MDT team would meet with family members quarterly to discuss their loved ones' plan of care and any concerns they may have; often, I observed family members leaving these meetings feeling confused, overwhelmed, or dissatisfied because they were unsure of the right questions to ask in order to achieve the desired outcomes.

"Enough is Enough."

I am committed to helping as many people as possible by sharing my insights on long-term care facilities. Through this series, I aim to connect with and support numerous individuals who share the same objective: achieving better care in a secure environment. I am thrilled to launch Nursing Home Secrets Volume One as the first step in helping you with this journey. **"Your Voice will be Heard."**

I would like to take a moment to thank you for purchasing this book. Prepare to discover a valuable resource that often been overlooked. This hidden gem provides crucial insights to assist you in addressing your challenges and concerns more profoundly.

Copyright

Disclaimer

Much of the publication is based on personal experience and the stories in this book reflect the author's recollection of events, thoughts, and opinions. The dialogue has been recreated from memory; Some names, locations, and identifying characteristics have been changed to protect the privacy of those depicted; any resemblance to actual persons living or dead or actual events is purely coincidental.

Any information contained on eBooks, books, audio-books, all social media platforms, or any form of communication, is provided for educational and informational purposes only and is not to be relied upon as a legal, medical or health professional opinion whatsoever.

All content mentioned does not constitute professional advice and is not guaranteed to be accurate, complete, reliable, current or error free. No liability is assumed for losses or damages due to the information provided. You are responsible for your own choices, actions, and results. You Hear Me Now LLC, the author and publisher assume no responsibility for errors or omissions in the contents of eBooks, books, audio-books, all social media platforms, or any form of communication.

In no event shall You Hear Me Now LLC, the author and/or the publisher be liable for any special direct, indirect, consequential, or incidental damages or any damages whatsoever, whether in an action of contracts, negligence, or other tort, arising out of or in connection with the use of the contents of the information provided. You should use this information as you see fit and at your own risk. Your particular situation may not be exactly suited to the examples illustrated and you should adjust your use of the information and recommendations accordingly.

Any trademarks, service marks, product names or named features contained in eBooks, books, and audio-books are assumed to be the property of their respective owners and are used only for reference. There is no implied endorsement if You Hear Me Now LLC, the author and/or publisher uses one of these terms.

Note:

Please consult a medical professional or healthcare provider if seeking medical advice, diagnosis, or treatment. For specific legal guidance consult with an attorney or from a qualified lawyer regarding your situation.

New Surveillance Law

Surveillance

Esther's Law went into effect on March 23, 2022

Esther's Law is an Ohio law that allows nursing home resident's and their representatives to install electronic monitoring devices in their rooms. Only residents, their representatives, law enforcement's, or others permitted by the resident or their representatives can view or listen to the device.

The law addresses the residents rights to dignity and privacy where there is a roommate involved, and places requirements on the facility to make reasonable accommodations. Residents living with others must get permission from their roommate or their representative before using an electronic , monitoring device in their room.

Facilities can't deny admission, discharge, discriminate, or retaliate against residents for installing devices. They also can't obstruct, tamper with, or destroy the devices or recordings.

Special Note:

The law is named after Esther Piskor whose son Steve Piskor installed a hidden camera in her room to document abuse by nursing home staff.

For more information about installing electronic monitoring devices, contact your state Long-Term Care Ombudsman Program.

Esther's Law

If you haven't had the chance to watch the video and learn about Esther's Law, I encourage you to listen to Esther Piskor's story and her son Steve Piskor's quest for justice on her behalf.

Regina's Corner

"My Thoughts, My Opinion"

It is so important to observe and document any sudden changes your loved one is experiencing, such as agitation, being withdrawn, unwanted touching (a hug), and unreported bruises, just to name a few.

If you notice any unexplained changes in your loved one's behavior, reach out to the director of nursing or the social worker. Inquire whether they have a significant change care plan in place and, if so, request to know its contents. If they do not have such a plan, ask for an explanation. Nursing homes are required to notify you of any significant changes in your loved one's condition, regardless of whether the changes are positive or negative. If your loved one experiences a notable change, it may be necessary to update their care plan to effectively address the issue.

To report suspected abuse in a nursing home or assisted living facility or by staff of a home care agency, call the State Ombudsman's Office toll-free at 1-800-282-1206, or contact their regional long-term care ombudsman program.

Contents

Organizational Structures

Nursing homes typically have organizational charts to help define the management of staff and to show how different positions and departments relate to each other. The chart structure may include the company owner, followed by the administrators, directors, and other employees.

If you experience any issues with any department managers bring them to the attention of the administrator. Make sure to keep a record of your communications regarding the issue, including who you spoke with, the time and date of the conversation, and your reasons for believing it was not resolved.

If you do not receive any response from the administrator reach out to your State Long-Term Care Ombudsman for support.

SPECIAL NOTE:

All fifty states the District of Columbia, Puerto Rico and Guam have a long-term care ombudsman program.

BE PREPARED

Roles and Responsibilities

Understanding the roles and responsibilities of nursing home staff is cruicial as it enables you to grasp how each team member contributes to delivering services that enhance your loved one's quality of life and well-being in long-term care facilities.

This section will provide a summary of the following departments:

Nursing
Dietary
Other Departments
Activities
Maintenance
Housekeeping
Laundry
Social Services
Therapy Department
Bed Holds
Readmission

Equipped with this knowledge, you will be better prepared to advocate for your loved one's needs and to address any concerns or issues related to their care.

Chapter 1

Nursing Department

Diverse Roles and Numerous Responsibilities

- Director of Nursing (DON), (RN)
- Registered Nurse (RN)
- Licensed Practical Nurse (LPN)
- Nursing Assistant (CNA) or (STNA)
- Wound Care Nurse (RN)
- Assisted Living Nurse

Director of Nursing

A Director of Nursing (DON) in a nursing home is responsible for overseeing and managing the nursing staff and the overall nursing care provided to the residents.

Some of the key responsibilities of a DON include:

- Developing and implementing nursing policies and procedures to ensure high quality resident care.
- Monitoring and analyzing nursing documentation, staffing ratios, and incident reports.
- Provide clinical leadership and ongoing training.
- Collaborate with the medical director, and other department managers to address resident needs.

Regina's Corner

'My Thoughts, My Opinion"

In my experience working in long-term care, the DON served as the second in command, collaborating closely with the administrator. The DON was in charge of ensuring that all staff were properly trained in infection control, Alzheimer's care, and various other policies and procedures across all departments.

Registered Nurse (RN)

The RN plays a vital role in managing resident care and supervising nuring staff in a nursing home.

The RN responsibilities may include:

- Assess residents' health conditions
- Administer medications and treatments such as, IV therapy, and tube feeding
- Coordinate with doctors regarding changes in resident status
- Responsible for supervising LPNs and other nursing staff, ensuring proper care is given
- Monitoring vital signs and documenting all care provided
- Work closely with other healthcare team members

RNs must ensure compliance with facility protocols and maintain accurate medical records.

Licensed Practical Nurse (LPN)

LPN's in a nursing home provides direct hands on resident care
under the supervision of an RN.

Their daily responsibilities may include:

- Administering medications
- Performing treatments and routine procedures such as catheter care, and basic wound dressing changes.
- Monitoring residents' conditions throughout their shift
- Supervise and direct CNAs and STNAs (Nursing Assistance)

LPNs maintain documentation of all care provided, assist with resident transfers, and communicate with families abcut basic care needs.

Nursing Assistant

A State Tested Nursing Assistant (STNA) and a Certified Nursing Assistant (CNA) perform essentially the same job duties in a nursing home; the main difference is the terminology used by different states. **For example, Ohio uses the term STNA, while most other states use CNA.** Both roles require completion of state approved training programs, passing a state competency exam, and maintaining state certification.

Nursing Assistants:

- Assist residents with activities of daily living (ADLs) including bathing, dressing, grooming, toileting, and eating.
- Help residents with mobility by assisting them in and out of chairs, bed, transferring to wheelchairs, and walking.
- They may take and record vital signs
- Record food and fluid intake
- Monitor residents for any changes in condition, reporting concerns to the nurses
- They make beds, keep residents' rooms clean and help maintain a safe environment

Nursing assistants role is fundamental to ensuring residents receive proper personal care while maintaining dignity and comfort.

Wound Care Nurse

Do all nursing homes have Wound Care Nurses? **NO**

A wound care nurse in a nursing home specializes in treating and preventing various types of wounds, with a focus on pressure ulcers, diabetic ulcers, surgical wounds, and other chronic wounds.

They perform:

- Comprehensive wound assessments
- Develop treatment plans
- Provide specialized wound care treatments
- Document wound healing progress through measurements, photographs, and detailed notes
- Collaborate with physicians

Wound nurses play a crucial role in preventing wounds by identifying high risk residents, implementing preventive measures, and educating staff about proper positioning, skin care, and early detection of skin breakdown.

Not all nursing homes have wound care nurses, but they should have a system in place to ensure that wounds are assesses and treated appropriately.

Wound care is important because improper care can lead to complications like infections, delayed healing, amputation and can cause pain and discomfort.

Nursing homes can implement a wound care program to ensure proper care for their residents.

Assisted Living Nurse

Assisted living nurses care for more independent residents who need minimal assistance, focusing mainly on medication management, and health monitoring with fewer regulatory requirements.

They work with lower nurse-to-resident ratios and emphasize supporting resident independence and quality of life.

Check with your assisted living community on thier policy for nurses and CNAs floor coverage.

Assisted living facilities may have LPNs or RNs on call, but they aren't required to be onsite every day.

Ask for their emergency procedure at night in case of a fire, tornado, falls, etc.

Nursing Department Summary

As highlighted in chapter one, nursing homes utilize a diverse range of licensed nursing professionals to deliver continuous care for their residents. Together, this interdisciplinary nursing team works to ensure nursing home residents receive the comprehensive care and support they require.

Other nurses in nursing homes not mentioned is, MDS (Minimum Data Set) Nurse and Nurse Practitioner.

Reminder: The Director of Nursing (DON) is responsible for managing the nursing department. The Registered Nurse (RN) supervises the Licensed Practical Nurse (LPN), who in turn oversees the nursing aides (CNAs), (STNAs).

Regina's Corner

My Thoughts, My Opinion"

If you encounter any issues with a nurse aide (nursing assistance), report it to the unit nurse on duty for that shift. Be sure to document detailed information, including whom you reported to, the specific issue or concern, the time and date of the report or incident, and the aides name.

Chapter 2

Dietary Department

- Dietitian
- Hydration
- Dehydration
- Weighing Resident's
- Weight Loss
- Weight Gain
- Weight Loss and Gain Summary
- Kitchen

Dietitian

Dietitian in nursing homes play a vital role in maintaining residents' health and quality of life by managing their nutritional care.

They look at residents eating patterns, allergies, therapeutic adjustments, food preferences, even religious beliefs.

Dietitians assess each resident's nutritional needs, develop personalized meal plans that account for medical conditions, medications, allergies, and swallowing difficulties, and **monitor residents' weight and nutritional status.**

Dietitians collaborate with nursing staff, physicians, and food service teams to ensure proper implementation of therapeutic diets, texture modifications, and dietary restrictions. They also provide nutrition education, address malnutrition concerns, manage tube feedings, and make recommendations for nutritional supplements. Additionally, dietitians participate in care planning meetings, **document nutritional interventions,** and ensure compliance with federal and state regulations regarding dietary services in long-term care facilities.

Hydration

Hydration

Hydration is critically important in nursing homes as older adults are particularly vulnerable to dehydration due to decreased thirst sensation, medication, and physical limitations that may make it difficult to drink independently. Proper hydration is essential for preventing serious complications such as urinary tract infections, confusion, falls, kidney problems, and hospitalizations.

Nursing home staff must actively monitor residents' fluid intake, offer drinks regularly throughout the day, provide assistance with drinking when needed, and recognize early signs of dehydration like dry mouth, dark urine, or changes in mental status.

Many facilities implement hydration programs that include scheduled drink rounds, tracking fluid intake, offering a variety of beverages, using adaptive drinking equipment when necessary, and educating both staff and residents about the importance of adequate fluid intake. During hot weather or illness, hydration becomes even more crucial, requiring increased vigilance and intervention from the care team to maintain residents' well-being.

Dehydration

Prevention Strategy

Staying hydrated is crucial for nursing home residents' health and well-being. With the right strategies, dehydration can be effectively prevented. You can speak to the Director of Nursing (DON) or the Dietitian.

Questions to ask and documents to obtain:

-Ask what is their hydration protocol?

-Ask for a copy of the policy and procedures for residents' hydration needs.

-What is the hydration protocol for residents'on nector, honey, or spoon-thickened liquids during and between meals?

-How do staff and nurse aides provide fluides between meals?

-Do they document fluid intake that is provided to residents in their rooms between meals

-Are the staff trained to recognize the signs of dehydration and respond appropriately?

-What interventions are currently in place for your loved one to help prevent dehydration, and their rehydration plan.

Everytime you visit, check to see if a freshwater pitcher is in the room and document what shift you were there. The water pitchers are supposed to be changed every shift.

Once you receive this information, you can use it with your hidden gem "provided in this guide book" to take action for any concerns you may have with this issue.

WEIGHT

Weighing Resident's

Most nursing homes use specialized wheelchair scales that can accommodate both the resident and their wheelchair.

The process typically involves the standard process for weighing wheelchair-bound residents:

1. Rolling the wheelchair onto the platform scale
2. Weighing both the resident and wheelchair together
3. Subtracting the wheelchair's weight (tare weight) from the total to get the resident's actual weight

There are two main types of scales used:

Platform scales - These are flat, ramp-style scales that allow the wheelchair to be rolled directly onto them. Many have handrails for safety.

Roll-on/roll-off scales - These are built into the floor so they're level with the ground, making it even easier to wheel resident's on and off.

To ensure accuracy:

-The wheelchair's empty weight is usually recorded and kept on file.
-Staff typically weigh residents at the same time of day.
-The scale is zeroed before each use
-Residents remain wearing similar clothing for consistency

For residents who can't use wheelchair scales, some facilities also use celing lift scales or specialized bed scales, but wheelchair scales are the most common method.

Weight Loss or Gain

WEIGHT LOSS

Weight loss in nursing homes is a serious concern that can indicate underlying health issues, neglect, or inadequate care. Common causes include depression, difficulty eating independently, dental problems, medication side effects, dysphagia (swallowing difficulties), dementia-related feeding issues, and sometimes undiagnosed medical conditions.

Staff shortages can lead to rushed mealtimes where residents don't receive adequate assistance with eating, while some residents may experience decreased appetite due to social isolation or institutional food quality. **Federal regulations require nursing homes to monitor residents' weight and intervene if there's a, loss of 5% or more in 30 days, 7.5% percent loss of body weight in 90 days or 10% in a 180 days, as significant weight loss can increase the risk of infections, pressure ulcers, falls, and other complications.**

Interventions typically include dietary modifications, nutritional supplements, assistance with feeding, treating underlying medical conditions, and monitoring food and fluid intake.

WEIGHT GAIN

Weight gain in nursing homes is a significant concern that can negatively impact residents' health and quality of life, often resulting from limited mobility, medication side effects (particularly from antipsychotics and steroids), fluid retention, hypothyroidism, or depression. Institutional settings may contribute to weight gain through reliance on high-calorie, processed foods, limited physical activity options, and the use of food as a source of comfort or entertainment.

Some residents may experience unintentional weight gain due to decreased metabolism associated with aging and inactivity, while others might overeat due to boredom or emotional issues.

Excess weight can exacerbate existing health conditions, increase the risk of pressure ulcers, make tranfers more difficult for staff, and complicate medical procedures.

Management typically involves dietary modifications, increase physical activity when possible, medication reviews, and addressing underlying psychological factors, though care must be taken to maintain quality of life while promoting healthy weight maintenance.

WEIGHT SUMMARY

Key questions to ask nursing home staff if you notice concerning weight changes in your loved one:

- How frequently are they weighed?
- What percentage of their meals are they consuming?
- Do they require assitance with eating, and are they receiving it?
- How much time are they allotted to finish their meals?
- What interventions are currently in place for weight management?
- What is the plan to address this weight change?
- Are there any progress notes regarding their eating habits?
- Ask to see their weight records?

Make sure to document these discussions and regularly follow up on any interventions that were promised.

KITCHEN

Kitchen

Nursing home kitchen responsibilities center around providing safe, nutritious meals while meeting strict health regulations and individual dietary needs. The kitchen staff must prepare three daily meals plus snacks, following therapeutic diet orders (pureed, diabetic, low sodium, etc.) and individual preferences documented in care plans. They maintain precise temperature controls for food safety, follow HACCP (Hazard Analysis Critical Control Points) guidelines, and keep detailed documentation of meal production and temperatures. **Kitchen staff must accommodate texture modifications, handle food allergies, and coordinate with nursing staff about residents' eating abilities and restrictions.** They're responsible for inventory management, ordering supplies, meal planning, and maintaining a clean, sanitized kitchen environment.

The dietary manager typically oversees menu planning with registered dietitians, ensures compliance with state and federal regulations, manages staff schedules, and coordinates special events or holiday meals.

Food service must operate seven days a week, three hundred and sixty five days a year, with backup plans for emergencies.

Dietary Summary

If you have concerns about the food being served, discuss alternatives with the kitchen manager. For any issues related to the diet plan , first consult the Dietitian and then reach out to the DON.

- Consult with the dietitian or unit nurse regarding your loved one's nutritional care plan to pinpoint any possible issues.
- Check with the unit nurse about any adjustments to their diet or alterations in eating habits.
- Ensure you participate in assisting them with menu selections if they need help choosing meals.
- Inquire if there is an alternative menu available.
- If you notice any weight flucuations in your loved one, feel free to ask questions.
- Confirm whether they have received their menu selections.

Always ensure that you document the date and time when you reported any issues, the person you spoke to, and their response. If the food-related problems continue, feel free to address your concerns directly with the administrator.

Chapter 3

Other Departments

Activities
Maintenance
Housekeeping
Laundry

One department that needs to be mentioned is the business office.

The business office handles all financial and administrative matters for residents, They manage billing and payments, work with insurance companies and Medicare/Medicaid, help residents and families understand their payment options and financial responsibilities, and maintain residents' accounts. They also process admissions paperwork, handle medical records documentation, and assist with questions about insurance coverage or payment plans. The business office serves as a key liaison between residents, their families, and various financial institutions or healthcare programs to ensure smooth financial operations during the resident's stay.

ACTIVITIES

Activities

If you find a facility that invests in the importance of developing a strong life enrichment program, I must say you have selected an excellent place for your loved one's well-being.

Regina's Corner
"My Experience, My Opinion"

Participating in activities help improve residents' mental well-being and can eliminate depression and social isolation. Activities give structure to the day, which give them a sense of purpose and help them pass the time away.

Unfortunately, the activities department suffers the most budget cuts and very limited on staffing.

Activity Director

Activity Directors in nursing homes, memory care and assisted living facilities play a vital role in maintaining residents' quality of life. Here are their key responsibilities:

1. **Program Planning and Impementation**

- Organize daily recreational activities like bingo, arts and crafts, and music sessions.
- Plan special events and holiday celebrations.
- Arrange religious services and spiritual activities.
- Coordinate exercise programs suitable for seniors.

2. **Social Engagement**

- Facilitate group discussions and social gatherings.
- Organize movie screenings and book clubs.
- Coordinate visits from volunteers and entertainers
- Plan outings when possible (weather and health permitting)

3. **Therapeutic Activities**

- Work with healthcare staff to provide activities that support physical and cognitive health.

- Organize memory care activities for residents with dementia.
- Conduct reminiscing therapy.
- Lead gentle exercise classes

4. Administrative Duties

- Assess residents' interests and capabilities.
- Document participation and engagement.
- Manage activity budgets.
- Train and supervise activity assistants.
- Ensure compliance with care regulations.

5. Individual Support

- Create personalized activity plans for residents.
- Help maintain connections with family through technology.
- Provide one-on-one activities for less mobile residents.
- Identify when residents might need additional support.

Activity Issues

If you're facing challenges with your loved one not engaging in activities, consider reaching out to the Activity Director:

- Inquire about your loved one's participation history and the frequency of refusals.
- Discuss their care plan, focusing on the goals and interventions related to activity involvement.
- Share your loved one's preferences for various activities.
- If they are in a wheelchair, ask whether the nursing aides assist in bringing them to the activities.

To assist, review the activity calendar each month and highlight events they would like to join. This allows the activity team to stress the importance of helping them prepare for participation. **Sometimes, residents may want to join an activity but end up resting after a meal. Unfortunately, if no one helps them up until the next shift, they might miss out on what they wanted to attend.**

Engaging in activities within a nursing home is crucial, as it can enhance residents' quality of life in numerous ways, including mental well-being, physical health, social interaction, cognitive function, and a feeling of normalcy.

If you notice your loved one feeling isolated or less active than before, collaborate with the Activity Director and Social Worker to ensure their social needs are addressed.

Ultimately, the primary objective for all residents is to enhance their quality of life, providing them with meaning and purpose.

MAINTENANCE

Maintenance Issues

Residents can experience maintenance issues related to:

- Plumbing problems.
- The temperture in their room or other parts of the building.
- Inadequate lighting in hallways and rooms.
- Damaged flooring and walls.
- Problem with ramps and broken handrails.
- Issues with equipment like broken wheelchairs or medical devices.

"All of which can affect residents, safety, and comfort."

Poor maintenance can lead to hazards like falls, infections, and discomfort due to extreme temperatures. Report maintenance issues to the department manager, administrator, or ombudsman.

If you encounter any maintenance issues, inform the floor nurse in that unit. If the problem persists, escalate the matter to the maintenance manager, followed by notifying the administrator.

HOUSEKEEPING

Housekeeping

Maintaining a clean building is a collective effort; it is not solely the duty of housekeeping, which focuses on deep cleaning. Everyone plays a part in this responsibility. Nurse aides should tidy up after assisting residents with toileting. disposing of adult briefs, changing trash, and placing soiled items on appropriate containers.

The kitchen needs to clean up spills in the dining room, mop the floor, vacuum the carpet and change tablecloths. Other staff members can help by picking items off the floor in hallways and throwing away empty containers you may see.

Regina's Corner

"My Experience, My Opinion"

With over twenty years of experience working with long-term care facilities, I can confidently say that they were all well-maintained and had pleasant odors-not the kind that tries to mask unpleasant smells like urine.

Housekeeping Issues

Housekeeping staff play a crucial role in cleaning and disinfecting residents' rooms, ensuring the facility remains sanitary to prevent the spread of disease by sanitizing entryways, doors, and furniture.

They also manage supplies such as bathroom tissue, paper towels, and hand soap, while ensuring a safe environment by keeping floors clean.

Key questions to consider:

- Is there an infection control protocol in place at the facility?
- How can residents' report their cleaning needs?
- Is your loved one's room included in a deep cleaning schedule, and how often does it occur?
- Who is responsible for deep cleaning and sanitizing the wheelchairs?

If you encounter any issues, you can express your concerns directly to the department manager, the facility administrator, and then Ombudsman.

Laundry Issues

Family members have often expressed their frustrations about loved ones' clothing and blankets being lost, shrunk, or damaged.

Preventive Strategies:

- Check if your facility has a policy regarding lost items.
- Retain receipts for all your purchases.
- Maintain an inventory of personal belongings.
- Label the inside of clothing and bedding with your family members' names.

If you encounter problems with missing clothing, approach the department manager. **Should your concerns remain unresolved, reach out to the social worker or business manager to discuss reimbursement options.**

Assisted Living Laundry

-Most assisted living facilities offer laundry services as a standard part of their care.

-Inquire whether the nursing aides help with laundry or if the facility's housekeeping and laundry department handles these needs, and find out how frequently this service is available.

SERVICES

Chapter 4

Services

Social Services
Therapy Services
Therapy Discharge

Special Note:

Assisted Living facilities are not federally regulated, so they are not required to have a social **Worker.** The center for Medicare and Medicaid Servces (CMS) requires nursing homes with more than 120 beds to have at least one full-time social worker.

"ALL ARE REQUIRED TO PROVIDE SOCIAL SERVICES"

Social Services

Social workers in nursing homes serve as essential advocates and support systems for residents and their families, helping to ensure both emotional well-being and proper care coordination.

They conduct psychosocial assessments, help residents and families adjust to facility life, ***mediate conflicts, and coordinate discharge planning when applicable. Social service workers assist with advance directives, financial concerns, and accessing community resources or benefits like Medicare and Medicaid.***

Social workers also provide counseling services to help residents cope with loss, depression, and anxiety, while facilitating support groups and social activities to combat isolation. They serve on interdisciplinary care teams, helping to ensure resident's rights are protected and their preferences are respected in care decisions. Additionally, ***they investigate and address any concerns about abuse or neglect,*** coordinate family meetings, and help maintain connections between residents and their loved ones. Their role extends to crisis intervention, end-of-life care planning, and ensuring compliance with social service regulations in long-term care settings.

Social services have a vital support role in therapy by:

1. Coordinating care between different healthcare providers, therapists, and families.
2. Providing emotional and psychological support to residents during their therapy journey.
3. Helping residents adjust to facility life and cope with changes in their health status.
4. Addressing barriers to therapy participation (like depression or family concerns).
5. Ensuring residents' rights and preferences are respected in their treatment plans.
6. Facilitating communication between residents, families, and the healthcare team.
7. Connecting residents with additional resources and support services as needed.

These services help create a more comprehensive care approach that supports both the physical and emotional aspects of therapy and recovery.

Therapy Department

Therapy Important Information

Physical Therapy

Occupational Therapy

Speech Therapy

Respiratory Therapy

Therapy Medicare Coverage

Here's important information about Medicare coverage for skilled nursing facility (SNF) therapy services:

Qualifying Requirements:

-Must have a qualifying three day minimum hospital stay
-Must need skilled therapy services daily
-Must be admitted to the Skilled Nursing Facility (SNF) within thirty days of hospital discharge
-Doctor must certify skilled nursing care is needed

Coverage Periods:

- **Days 1-20:** Medicare pays 100%
- **Days 21-100:** Patient pays daily coinsurrance ($204.00 in 2024), Medicare covers remainder
- **Beyond 100 days:** No Medicare coverage for that benefit period

Types of Covered Therapy:

-Physical Therapy
-Occupational Therapy
-Speech Therapy
-Respiratory Therapy when needed

Important Notes:

- Therapy must be reasonable and necessary for condition
- Progress must be documented and measurable
- Coverage can stop before one hundred days if patient plateaus or no longer needs skilled care
- A new benefit period can begin after sixty days without inpatient care
- Must be making progress toward goals

Not Covered:

- ***Long-term custodian care***
- ***Room and board once skilled needs end***
- ***Personal care only services***
- ***Therapy maintenance without skilled need***

Documentation Requirements:

-Physician orders and certification
-Therapy evaluations and progress notes
-Daily skilled notes
-Weekly progress summaries

It's important to note that coverage decisions are made based on medical necessity and progress, not solely on the availability of benefit days.

The aim of therapy is to empower you to become strong enough to return home safely.

Physical Therapy

Physical therapy in skilled nursing facilities provides specialized rehabilitation services to residents recovering from surgery, injury, or illness. Licensed physical therapists and assistants work with patients to improve mobility, strength, balance, and functional independence through individualized exercise programs, gait training, and therapeutic modalities. Sessions typically occur multiple times per week in a dedicated therapy gym equipped with specialized equipment like parallel bars, stairs, and therapeutic exercise machines.

The goal is to help residents regain their highest possible level of physical function so they can either return home safely or maintain their current level of independence within the facility.

Occupational Therapy

Occupational therapists in skilled nursing facilities help residents maintain or regain independence is daily living activities. They evaluate and treat residents' abilities to perform tasks like dressing, bathing, eating, and grooming, often adapting techniques or recommending equipment to compensate for physical or cognitive limitations. They also address upper body strength, fine motor skills, and cognitive function through therapeutic activities and exercises.

OTs work closely with residents who have experienced strokes, injuries, or degenerative conditions, creating personalized treatment plans that focus on maximizing function and quality of life while preventing further decline.

Speech Therapy

Speech therapists (also called speech-language pathologists) in nursing homes **help residents with swallowing problems, communication difficulties, and cognitive issues. They evaluate and treat swallowing disorders (dysphagia) to prevent choking and aspiration, help residents who have trouble speaking due to strokes or other conditions, and work on memory and cognitive skills.** They also assist residents who use communication devices or need modified diets for safe eating. The therapists often collaborate with nursing staff to implement strategies for safe feeding and effective communication with residents.

Respiratory Therapy

Respiratory therapy in skilled nursing homes provide specialized care for residents with breathing difficulties, chronic respiratory conditions, and those requiring ventilator support or oxygen therapy. Licensed respiratory therapists work alongside nurses and physicians to assess patients, develop and implement treatment plans, momitor oxygen levels, manage breathing techniques, medication delivery through inhalers or nebulizers, and airway clearance methods. This specialized care is particularly crucial for residents with conditions like COPD and pneumonia, helping to prevent hospitalizations and maintain optimal respiratory function in the long-term care setting.

TRANSFER & DISCHARGE

Therapy Discharge

WHEN THERAPY IS OVER

Before the nursing home proposes a transfer or a discharge, a facility must identify and try to meet the resident's individual medical, nursing, and psychosocial needs. They would do so by formulating and implementing an individualized care plan designed to meet those needs. Many of the permissible reasons for transfer or discharge can be addressed through assessment and care planning, making tranfer or discharge unnecessary.

Because most nursing homes provide fairly complex care for sick residents, rarely the facility cannot find a way to provide adequate care for the resident or to keep the resident and others safe with the use of a good assessment and care plan.

When a resident reaches a stable state-meaning they are no longer making progress-Medicare may discontinue coverage for therapy services. Therefore, it's important to discuss discharge planning as soon as your loved one begins therapy at a skilled nursing facility.

The therapy department will begin discussions about discharging or transferring a resident before they reach one hundred days if no progress is evident.

"SUBMIT YOUR MEDICAID APPLICATION WITHOUT DELAY"

Reform Law

Aging.ohio.gov (Ohio Department of Aging)

The nursing home reform law of 1987 prohibits nursing homes from transferring or discharging a resident unless it can establish that one other permissible reason for transfer or discharge exists:

1. The nursing home is unable to deliver sufficient care for the resident.
2. The resident's health has improved to a level where nursing home care is no longer necessary.
3. The safety of individuals within the facility is at risk.
4. The health of others in the facility would be compromised.
5. The resident has not made payments for care despite receiving reasonable and appropriate notice.

However, the facility cannot evict a resident who is awaiting Medicaid eligibility and should collaborate with other state agencies to secure payment if the resident's funds are being held by a family member or another individual, or of the facility has ceased operations.

Contact the Long-Term Care Ombudsman Program if you are concerned about plans for transfer or discharge from a nursing home. **The ombudsman is empowered by law to advocate for nursing home residents.**

TRANSFER & DISCHARGE

Notification
Time Limits
Your Rights

Transfer or Discharge Notice

NOTIFICATION

If a resident is to transfer or discharge, the facility must record the reason for transfer in the resident clinical record. They must also notify the resident and the residents family member, guardian, or legal representative in writing. The notice must include:

- The reason for the transfer or discharge.
- The location to which the resident will be moved.
- The date of transfer or discharge.
- Information about the residents right to appeal to the state concerning the transfer or discharge, with the name, address, and telephone number of the state long-term care ombudsman.

The location the resident will be moved to must be specific, appropriate, available, and agreeable to taking the resident.

Time Limits

The law requires that a nursing home must inform the resident and the resident's family member, guardian or legal representative about a transfer or discharge at least thirty days in advance:

- The nursing home must provide discharge planning and sufficient preparation and orientation to residents being transferred or discharged.
- The law guarantees the right of the resident or responsible family member to participate in planning care and treatment, which should include choosing a new place to live.
- The nursing home should prepare an orientation, such as a visit to the new home, and ensure a safe arrival.
- The resident should know where they are going.
- The facility should inform the new facility about the residence needs, preferences, and habits.
- The nursing home should ensure possessions aren't lost in the moving process and any personal funds are given to the resident or transferred to a new account.

Your Rights

The Nursing Home Resident Protection Amendment of 1999 is a law that protects the rights of nursing home residents.

Nursing homes must continue to provide care for Medicaid residents even if they stop participating in Medicaid.

Nursing homes cannot transfer or discharge residents because they voluntarily stopped participating in Medicaid. Residents have the right to appeal a transfer or discharge decision.

Complaints and Appeals

A resident has the right to appeal the facilities decision to transfer or discharge him or her. The transfer or discharge notice must include information about how to request a hearing, the resident's right to use legal counsel or other spokesperson at the hearing, and the mailing address and telephone number of the state long-term care ombudsman. A complaint may also be filed with the state survey agency.

Residents can refuse to be transferred from one certified level of care to another.

Example: A facility requires a bed for a new admission, but the nursing unit is full. Consequently, they opt to transfer Mr. D to the Alzheimer unit to free up his room for the new patient. Mr. D begins to express his concerns and inquires about the reason for his move. By the end of the day, Mr. D was promptly returned to his original room.

Residents and their families must be notified before a resident room or roommate changes.

Bed Holds

Bed Holds and Readmissions

Here's a concise overview of the key regulations regarding bed holds and readmissions in nursing homes:

Bed Holds:

1. Medicaid requires states to have a bed hold policy but specifics vary by state.
2. Facilities must notify residents and or families about bed hold policies upon admission and before transfers.
3. Typically covers temporary hospital stays or therapeutic leave.
4. Duration varies by state (commonly 7-15 days)
5. Facilities may charge private pay residents to hold beds.

Readmission Rights:

1. Residents have the right to return to the first available bed in a semi-private room if:

-They were hospitalized

-Their needs can still be met by the facility

-They still require nursing home level care

2. **Medicaid eligible residents must be re-admitted to their previous room if available.**
3. **Facilities cannot require a new entrance fee for readmission.**

4. **Residents may be denied readmisssion only if they:**

-No longer need nursing home care

-Endanger health and or safety of others

-Have care needs the facility cannot meet

Bed Holds & Readmissions

Nursing homes must follow federal and state regulations regarding bed holds and readmissions. When residents are temporarily hospitalized, facilities must inform residents and their families about bed hold policies. While Medicaid requires states to have bed hold policies, private pay residents may be charged to maintain their bed.

Medicare does not pay for bed holds at all.

Medicaid coverage for bed holds varies by state-some states Medicaid programs will pay to hold a bed for a limited number of days (typically ranging from 5-15 days), while other states provide no Medicaid coverage for bed holds. You would need to check your specific state's Medicaid policy. **If you want the bed held and it's not covered by Medicaid in your state, you (or your family) would need to pay the facility's daily private rate to hold the bed during a hospital stay. The facility must inform you of these costs and policies in writing.**

Even without paying for a bed hold, Medicaid recipients still maintain their right to return to the first available bed in a semi-private room once they're ready to return from the hospital, as long as they remain Medicaid-eligible and meet the facility's level of care requirements.

Section One Summary

Roles and Responsibilities

Section one introduces you to the various departments that make up the framework of long-term care communities, providing concise descriptions to clarify their functions. Understanding who supervises or manages each department is essential, as it helps you grasp their impact on your loved one's quality of life. With this information, you'll be better prepared to address your concerns and issues with the right individual.

Requesting your facilities organizational chart will give you a better understanding whom to contact regarding any concerns.

Always keep your rights in mind when contemplating discharge or transfer to a different facility. If you run out of funds for therapy, there are options you can explore. Make sure to speak with the social worker or reach out to the Ombudsman to start the Medicaid application process as soon as possible.

Ombudsman is available in 50 states, the District of Columbia, Puerto Rico and Guam have a long-term care ombudsman program.

To find your state Ombudsman **example: (your state name) long-term care ombudsman hotline.**

"Utilize Your Resources"

KNOW THE SYSTEM

WHO IS WATCHING WHOM?

Assisted Living

Nursing Homes

Ombudsman

Annual and Complaint State Survey

Understanding Deficiency Citations

Summary

Know the System

KNOW THE SYSTEM
"WHO IS WATCHING WHOM"

Section two will provide an in-depth exploration of how nursing homes and assisted living facilities operate, with an emphasis on the regulations and survey processes that are essential to their functioning.

Nursing homes in the United States are heavily regulated at both the federal and state levels. At the federal level, the Centers for Medicare and Medicaid Services (CMS) sets the regulations and standards that nursing homes must meet in order to participate in the Medicare and Medicaid programs. These regulations cover areas such as resident rights, quality of care, nursing staffing levels, infection control, and food services.

In addition to the federal oversight, many states have their own supplementary nursing home regulations and survey processes. The specific requirements can vary across different states and localities.

Chapter 5

Assisted Living

Are there different regulations for Assisted Living Facilities (ALF) compared to Nursing Homes? **YES**

In the United States ALFs are overseen by state agencies rather than the federal government. This oversight includes requirements for licensing and certifications, as well as the frequency of inspections.

The National Center for Assisted Living (NCAL) releases an annual Assisted Living state regulatory review, which outlines the essential liicensing or certification requirements for assisted living facilities across each state.

Assisted Living State Regulatory Review:
This resource is valuable for understanding the standards that govern assisted living facilities in your state and provides detail on how state agencies license facilities that care for residents with **Alzheimer's or other forms of dementia.**

Assisted living facilities undergo inspections at least once every nine to fifteen months. Additionally, these facilities must make their most recent inspection report readily accessible to residents, family members, and their representatives.

Assisted Living Regulations

Assisted living facilities (ALFs) are primarily regulated at the state level, with significant variation in regulations between states, unlike nursing homes which have strong federal oversight.

Here's the breakdown:

State Level Regulation (Primary):
-State Department of Health/HumanServices
-State Department of Aging
-State Licensing Boards
-State Long-Term Care Ombudsman
-State Adult Care Licensure Departments

Key Differences from Nursing Homes:
-No federal oversight like the Center for Medicare and Medicaid Services (CMS)
-No federal funding through Medicare
-Less stringent regulations than nursing homes
-Varies significantly state by state
-Different licensing requirements by state

Typical State Oversight Areas:
-Staffing requirements

-Training standards
-Medication management
-Building safety codes
-Food service standards
-Emergency procedures
-Resident rights
-Admission and discharge criteria
-Service scope limitations

Additional Oversight:
-Local health departments
-Fire marshals
-Adult Protective Services
-Building safety inspectors
-Local zoning boards

Inspection Process:
-Annual state inspections
-Complaint investigations
-License renewal reviews
-Life safety code inspections
-Food service inspections

It is important to note that because regulation is primarily state based, there can be significant differences in standards, requirements, and quality oversight between different states.

Assisted Living

SURVEY INSPECTION

Here's a brief summary of the typical procedure for conducting surveys and inspections of assisted living facilities:

Licensing and Regulations:

-Each state licenses and regulates assisted living facilities, with unique laws and requirements.

-State agencies, such as the Department of Health or Department of Social Services, oversee these facilities.

Routine Surveys:

-Assisted living facilities are subject to regular, unannounced surveys or inspections, typically on an annual or every 2 year basis.

-State surveyors assess compliance with regulations related to resident care, staffing, facility upkeeping, and administration

Survey Process:

-Surveyors examine the facility's policies, procedures, and documentation.

-They interview staff, residents, and family members.

-Observations of the facility's operations, including meal service, activities, and medication management, are also conducted during their visits.

Deficiency Citations:

-When a facility is determined to be non-compliant with regulations, surveyors will issue deficiency citations.

-These citations specify the particular issues that the facility must address.

Plan of Corrections:

-The facility is required to submit a plan of correction to the state agency, outlining how it intends to rectify the identified deficiencies.

-Approval from the state is necessary before the facility can implement the required changes.

Follow-up Visits:

-The state agency may carry out follow-up visits to confirm the facility has resolved the cited deficiencies.

-Should the facility fail to address the issues, it could penalties, including fines or the potential suspension revocation of its license.

Public Reporting:

-The outcomes of assisted living facility surveys are generally made available to the public, often through state agency websites or databases.

-Consumers can utilize this information to evaluate the quality and compliance record of facilities when selecting an assisted living community.

This process is essential in ensuring that assisted living facilities uphold proper standards of care and safety for their residents.

Chapter 6

Nursing Home

"WHO IS WATCHING WHOM"

Nursing homes are regulated by multiple agencies at different levels of government:

Federal Level:

-Centers for Medicare and Medicaid Services (CMS)
-Department of Health and Human Services (HHS)
-Food and Drug Administration (FDA)
-Occupational Safety and Health Administration (OSHA)

State Level:

-State Department of Health
-State Licensing Boards
-State Long-Term Care Ombudsman
-State Survey Agencies (Conduct Inspections)
-State Medicaid Agencies

Additional Oversight:

-Joint Commission (If Accredited)
-Adult Protective Services
-State Attorney Generals Office
-Local Health Departments

Nursing Homes

Nursing home facilities are subject to extensive regulation by both federal and state agencies, with the Centers for Medicare and Medicaid Services (CMS) acting as the main federal authority.

They must adhere to numerous stringent regulations addressing various aspects such as residents rights, quality of care, staffing levels and safety standards.

State agencies carry out regular unannounced inspections (surveys) to verify compliance, and facilities **are required to report quality measures and staffing information to retain their licenses.**

Violations can lead to fines, lower ratings, or in serious cases, revocation of licenses. Facilities are evaluated on a five-star rating system through Medicare's nursing home compare website, which assesses health inspections, staffing levels, and quality measures.

The state's long-term care Ombudsman program offers additional oversight by advocating for residents' rights and addressing complaints, while Adult Protective Services and state licensing boards also play vital roles in ensuring the safety and quality of care for residents.

Regulations

Nursing homes are required to be in compliance with federal regulations to receive payment under Medicare or Medicaid.

Key Regulations:

-OBRA (Omnibus Budget Reconcilition Act) guidelines
-Federal and State nursing home regulations
-Life Safety Codes
-Health Insurance Portability and Accountability Act (HIPAA)
-Americans with Disabilities Act (ADA)

Inspection Process:

-Annual state surveys (unannounced)
-Complaint investigations
-Follow-up visits for violations
-Federal oversight surveys
-Quality measure reporting

Compliance Areas:

-Quality of care
-Staffing levels
-Residents rights
-Safety standards
-Infection control
-Food service
-Medication management
-Documentation requirements

Ombudsman

All 50 states the District of Columbia, Puerto Rico and Guam have a long-term care ombudsman program.

Ombudsman are advocates for nursing home and assisted living residents, who can help with complaints, resolve problems and educate consumers and long-term care providers about resident rights and good care practices. They can also help people understand their rights and access benefits.

The Administration on Aging, within the Department of Health and Human Services, administers the Long-Term Care Ombudsman Program. The program is mandated by the Older Americans Act, to advocate for improvements in long-term care and address complaints.

The program is managed by following entities:

-State long-term care (LTC) ombudsman program.

-National Consumer Voice for Quality Long-Term Care operates the National Ombudsman Resource Center (NORC).

-The National Association of Local Long-Term Care Ombudsman works closely with (NORC).

-National Association of State LTC Ombudsman Programs works closely with NORC.

Contact your state long-term care ombudsman program and

let them know about your concerns.

Chapter 7

Annual & Complaint State Survey

This chapter will offer you crucial insights into the procedures involved in an annual or complaint state survey inspection. Understanding this process is vital for you to know how long-term care facilities prevent citations and for you to gain a clearer perspective on what occurs when a complaint is filed.

Preparations Taking Places Behind the Scenes.

The annual survey in nursing homes typically occurs around the same time each year, with some facilities referring to this period as "The Window," anticipating the state's arrival for their yearly inspection.

To prepare, the facility may conduct a mock survey involving management from other locations within the company. This allows for a thorough inspection of all departments-such as Dietary, Activities, Maintenance, and Nursing, to identify potential issues, enabling each department to make necessary corrections before the actual survey/inspection.

A behind the scenes, when the state is present.

-Typically, visits last between three to five days. The administrator and director of nursing feeling a bit anxious after the third day.

-It is crucial for all managers to ensure their departments are fully staffed and ready, as the facility does not prioritize overtime.

-Managers from every department, along with behind-the-scenes staff, are required to be on the floor, responding to call lights and helping with meals. "Staff will be everywhere," and corporate representatives will also be available if needed.

-No member of the management team is permitted to leave for the day until the survey team has finished their work and leave the building.

The goal is to decrease all possibilities of receiving a citation "they call it an F-tag."

Annual Survey

When the state arrives at the facility, they will first meet with the administrator and the director of nursing to clarify whether their visit is fo a complaint investigation or an annual inspection.

On the initial day, the surveyors will be seated in a designated room provided by the facility, where they will request various documents.

The documents they may review include:

- Minutes from the Resident Council meetings.
- The nursing home's previous compliance records.
- Complaints filed against the nursing home.
- Fire and safety policies.
- Protocols related to resident care, abuse or injury, and emergency responses.
- Dietary practices.

After examining the documents, the surveyors will move throughout the facility, spending each day observing different departments, asking questions, and requesting additional documents as necessary. If they identify any issues during their observations, they will inquire further; If you cannot answer their questions, it is essential to find someone who can.

Upon completing their investigation, the surveyors will conduct what is known as an exit review. They will meet with the administrator and the director of nursing to discuss their findings from the investigation.

Regina's Corner

"My Thoughts, My Opinion"

No nursing home is flawless. The state surveyors will highlight any deficiencies they discover and allow the nursing home an opportunity to address them. Depending on the nature of the deficiencies, if the facility submits an action plan within the specified timeframe, they may avoid potential costly fines.

Complaint Survey

State surveyors look at the health and happiness of residents by reviewing the resident council minutes.

How often have you heard someone mention their intention to contact the state and file a complaint against a nursing home, assisted living, or memory care facility? The reality is that long-term care facilities have faced numerous inspections for complaints, making them quite accustomed to the process.

What to expect when you call and file a complaint with the state:

The state surveyors will convene with the administrator and the director of nursing to discuss the complaint. Following this, the surveyor will investigate the issue by requesting resident council minutes, reviewing documentation, and interviewing individuals related to the allegations. If the surveyor uncovers any discrepancies based on your complaint, they will allow the facility time to rectify the issue. Should the facility successfully address the problem during the investigation and before the exit review, the surveyor will categorize the allegations as unsubstantiated (not supported or proven by evidence), which means the facility will avoid incurring any costly fines.

A nursing home survey / inspection may be deemed unsubstantiated if the state surveyor concludes that the reported noncompliance did not result in actual harm to a resident.

"WHAT DOES THIS MEAN?"

The surveyor must uncover a significant issue for the facility to incur a serious penalty. This severe penalty, referred to as an Immediate Jeopardy (IJ), indicates that the facility has jeopardized the health and safety of its residents, potentially leading to serious injury, harm, impairment, or even death. An IJ can result in costs of up to $10,000 per day for the facility.

I'm not suggesting that the nursing home won't be cited for your complaint; however, when it comes to citations that result in fines, long-term care facilities often hire specialized consultants to address the specific issues cited. Their objective is to develop a corrective action plan to prevent expensive fines.

Nursing homes will go to great lengths to protect their financial interests. Always be prepared and have your notes and documentation ready when filing a complaint to support your case, as it will likely be contested, and the facility will have the opportunity to rectify any problems.

The cornerstone of your complaint lies in thorough documentation, which serves as your hidden gem. Ultimately, after the dust settles from annual inspection or a complaint, the facility tends to revert to its previous practices and routines.

Chapter 8

Understanding Deficiency Citations

This chapter will explain to you the deficiency citations that nursing homes, memory care and assisted living facilities can recieve durng their annual or complaint survey/inspection.

1. Quality of Care
-Pressure ulcer prevention/treatment failures
-Falls prevention issues
-Medication errors
-Poor infection control practices

2. Resident Rights
-Failure to respect dignity/preferences
-Privacy violations
-Inadequate grievance procedures

3. Environmental
-Unsanitary conditions

-Fire safety violations
Building maintenance issues

4. Staffing

-Inadequate nurse staffing levels
-Untrained personnel
-Poor supervision

5. Assessment & Care Planning

-Incomplete assessments
-Failure to update care plans
-Poor documentation

Each deficiency is rated by scope (isolated vs pattern vs widespread) and severity (minimal harm to immediate jeopardy). The most serious deficiencies can result in fines, required corrective actions, or even closure.

Isolation Scope Deficiency

Example of an isolated scope deficiency citation: During the annual survey on 7/23/22, one resident out of 25 was observed not receiving assistance with eating during lunch despite their care plan requiring feeding assistance. The resident care plan indicated they needed total assistance with meals due to right-sided weakness. The resident was observed picking at their food for 20 minutes while staff passed by multiple times without stopping to help. When interviewed, staff stated they were short-staffed that day and "must have missed" the resident. This resulted in the resident consuming less than 25% of their meal.

This would likely be cited as F676 (Activities of Daily Living) at a scope of "Isolated" since it affected one resident, with potential for minimal harm since it was one meal.

Pattern Scope Deficiency

Example of a Pattern scope deficiency citation: During the annual survey from 6/14 thru 6/18/2020, review of 30 resident records revealed 8 residents (27%) lacked complete fall risk assessments following their falls, while incident reports documented the falls occurred, the facility failed to conduct post-fall assessments per their policy.

Specifically:

-Three residents had no documented neurological checks after hitting their heads.

-Five residents had no environmental assessment to identify fall contributing factors.

-Four residents had no documented changes to their care plans after falls.

-Some residents had multiple missing assessments.

Interviews with nursing staff revealed inconsistent understanding of the facility's fall protocol. Two nurses stated they "weren't sure" when neurological checks were required, while another thought environmental assessments were "optional."

Review of three months of fall data showed this was'nt isolated. Approximately 30% of falls consistently lacked proper follow-up documentation.

This would likely be cited as F689 (Free of Accidents/Supervision) at Pattern scope since it represents a systemic breakdown in fall protocol affecting a significant number of residents across different units and shifts.

Widespread Scope Deficiency

Example of a Widespread scope deficiency citation:

During the annual survey 4/15 thru 4/19/2021, the facility failed to maintain required hot water temperatures between 100-120 degrees fahrenheit in all resident care areas. Temperature readings throughout the building showed consistently high temperatures between 128-135 degrees fahrenheit across all wings (A, B, C and D), affecting all 98 residents. Multiple residents complained of "too hot" water and staff were observed adding cold water to basins before providing care.

Maintenance logs showed no temperature monitoring for three months. The director of maintenance stated the main water heater's temperature regulator "hasn't worked right" sinceFebruary but hadn't been repaired due to "budget issues."

This would be cited as F689 (Safe Environment) at Widespread scope since it affects the entire resident population and all areas of the facility.

Deficiency Classification

In nursing home surveys/inspections, you have Minimal or Immediate Jeoparty classifications that indicates the level of harm.

Minimal Harm Deficiency

In nursing home surveys/inspections, "minimal harm" is a deficiency classification that indicates:

1. A violation of regulations was found.
2. The violation resulted in little to no actual harm to residents.
3. The potential for harm to residents was minimal.
4. The issue posed a very low risk to resident health and safety.

This is the lowest level of deficiency severity. Examples of minimal harm findings might include:

-Minor documentation errors.
-Slight delays in non-critical services.
-Minor enviromental issues that don't directly impact resident care.
-Small procedural deviations that don't affect resident outcomes.

Higher levels include:

-Potential for harm
-Actual harm
-Immediate jeopardy

Immediate Jeopardy Deficiency

Immediate Jeopardy (IJ) is the most serious deficiency level in nursing home, memory care and assisted living survey/inspections.

Here's what it means:

1. Definition:

-A situation causing or likely to cause serious injury, harm, impairment, or death to residents.

-Requires immediate intervention to prevent harm

2. Key Characteristics:

-Immediate threat to resident health or safety

-Requires rapid response and correction

-Often results in significant penalties

-May lead to termination from Medicare and Medicaid programs if not corrected

3. Common Examples:

-Failure to prevent or respond to abuse

-Serious medication errors

-Failure to monitor critial medical conditions

-Major infection control breaches

-Life safety code violations that could cause immediate harm

-Failure to provide emergency care

4. Consequences:

-Substantial fines (often thousands of dollars per day)
-Required immediate corrective action
-Possible temporary management
-Potential closure if not corrected
-Mandatory state monitoring
-Loss of federal funding if not addressed

YOUR HIDDEN GEM

RESIDENT COUNCIL AND FAMILY COUNCIL MINUTES

So, why is resident and family council your hidden gem?

Resident council minutes serve as your powerful tool for documenting concerns each month. Every department is obligated to address all the issues raised, ensuring that everyone's voice is heard. Resident council minutes is one of the first documents surveyors/inspectors ask for.

Chapter 9

Resident & Family Council

Resident council minutes are typically one of the first documents requested by state surveyors.

You have the right to establish and engage in Resident and Family Councils. Unfortunately, many family members overlook this valuable opportunity to collectively express concerns on a monthly basis.

In my two decades of experience in care facilities, I have yet to see a family council.

This chapter will summarize the significance of the Resident and Family Council as a valuable yet frequently overlooked resource. It embodies the essential documentation and serves as a vital voice that should be recognized and amplified.

RESIDENT COUNCIL

Resident Council Minutes

A comprehensive explanation of how resident council minutes can be valuable.

1. Voice for Residents

-Documents resident concerns, suggestions, and feedback directly from their perspective.

-Creates an official record of what matters most to the residents.

-Helps ensure resident preferences are heard and considered in facility decisions.

2. Quality Improvement

-Tracks recurring issues that need attention.

-Identifies trends in resident satisfaction or dissatisfaction.

-Provides documentation for implementing changes based on resident input

-Helps measure if previous concerns were adequately addressed.

3. Regulatory Compliance

-Demonstrates compliance with federal requirements for resident councils.

-Provides evidence of resident participation in facility decisions.

-Shows the facility's commitment to resident rights and engagement.
-**Helps during state surveys/inspections.**

4. Communication Tool

-Keeps staff informed about resident needs and preferences.
-Helps bridge communication between different departments.
-Provides updates to family members about facility activities.
-Creates transparency between residents and administration.

5. Problem Solving

-Documents proposed solutions to issues.
-Tracks the implementation of changes.
-Shows follow through on resident requests.
-Helps evaluate the effectiveness of interventions.

Management Response

The proper management response to Resident Council Minutes

Here's what management should do:

1. Review and Acknowledge

-Read all minutes thoroughly
-Document that management has reviewed the minutes
-Respond to all concerns within a reasonable timeframe (typically within 30 days per federal regulations)

2. Take Action

-Address any complaints or grievance raised
-Implement feasible suggestions from residents
-Make necessary changes to policies or procedures based on feedback
-Document all actions taken in response to concerns

3. Communicate Back

-Provide written responses to the resident council
-Explain what actions will be taken and timeframes
-If a request cannot be fulfilled, explain why
-Keep residents information of progress on ongoing issues

4. Documentation

-Maintain records of all minutes and responses
-Include actions taken and their outcomes
-**Keep these records available for state inspectors**
-Include relevant information in quality assurance meetings

5. Follow-Up

-Monitor implementation of any changes
-Ensure promised actions are completed
-Report back to the council on outcomes
-Address any new concerns that arise from changes

Unaddressed

What typically happens when state surveyors find unaddressed issues in resident council minutes during a nursing home survey/inspection:

Citation Process. The facility may receive a deficiency citation, typically under F-tag 565 (Resident/Family Group and Response). This indicates non-compliance with federal requirements to address and respond to resident council concerns.

Required Response; The nursing home must develop a Plan of Correction (POC).

They need to demonstrate how they will:

-Address the specific unresolved issues.
-Implement a system to track and respond to council concerns.
-Prevent similar oversights in the future.
-Monitor compliance going forward.

Potential Consequences, depending on severity:

-Civil monetary penalties
-Required in-service training
-More frequent monitoring
-Impact on the facility's rating
-In serious cases, it could affect Medicare and Medicaid certification.

Follow-Up

Surveyors will conduct follow-up visits to ensure:

-The identified issues have been resolved

-New processes are in place

-The facility is responding appropriately to council concerns

Guidance

While resident councils are primarily for residents themselves, family members can support these meetings in several important ways:

Supporting resident participation:
-Encourage and help your loved one attend meetings
-Assist with transportation to the meeting location if needed
-Help them prepare topics they'd like to discuss

Appropriate ways to participate:
-Ask the council president or facility staff about policies for family attendance.
-Attend only if invited by residents or if facility policies permit
-Respect that this is primarily a resident-led forum
-Speak only when invited to do so by residents

Indirect Support
-Help communicate council decisions to other family members.
-Follow up on action items that residents request help with.
-Advocate for implementing council recommendations.
-Share concerns through proper channels if residents request.

Alternate Involvement

-Join or form a separate Family Council if one exists.

-Attend open meetings when invited.

-Participate in joint resident-family events.

-Meet with facility administration separately regarding concerns.

Regina's Corner

"My Thoughts, My Opinion"

Memory Care Unit/Facility

Unfortunately, residents with Alzheimer's are not invited to participate in resident council meetings, even though they have the right to do so. The Memory care unit exemplifies the necessity of establishing a family council, where relatives can collaborate to ensure that their loved one's needs are addressed.

FAMILY COUNCIL

Family Council

COMMON FOCUS AREAS

Working with Facility Staff
-Maintain professional, collaborative relationships
-Document concerns and requests in writing
-Follow proper channels for grievances
-Acknowledge positive changes and improvements
-Share council achievements and goals

Quality of Care
-Staffing Levels
-Medical Care
-Personal Care
-Nutrition
-Activities

Quality of Life
-Physical environment
-Social activities
-Emotional support
-Cultural sensitivity
-Religious and spiritual needs

Administrative Issues

-Communication policies

-Visiting hours

-Billing practices

-Staff training

-Emergency procedures

Measuring Success

-Track resolution of identified issues

-Monitor membership growth and participation

-Survey members regularly

-Document positive changes in facility

-Maintain records of achievements

Remember, a successful Family Council focuses on systemic improvements rather than individual complaints, maintains confidentiality, and works constructively with facility management while maintaining its independence.

Resident & Family Council Summary

Keeping thorough records during visits to loved ones, neighbors, or friends in long-term care facilities can be exhausting but is incredibly important. This is why participating in the resident council is vital. The minutes from these meetings are typically the first documents inspectors request, acting as a guide for their evaluation, despite their comprehensive assessment of the entire facility. From these minutes, surveyors can determine which residents and family members to interview.

When lodging a complaint, it's crucial to remember that surveyors may interpret it as emotional rather than factual. Having access to the resident council minutes enables them to discern whether an issue is isolated, part of a larger trend, or widespread, and whether the facility has taken action to resolve these problems.

Meetings occur monthly, and surveyors can review up to a year's worth of council minutes to determine if issues are recurring.

If you are located far from your loved one's facility, consider checking with the Ombudsman about the possibility of conducting family council meetings through video conferencing. There is power in collective voices addressing common concerns and issues.

While complaints may arise from emotional responses, blending these feelings with factual information can create a meaningful difference.

Be sure to obtain a copy of the original draft of the council minutes and the finalized typed version.

Contact Your State Long-Term Care Ombudsman Program to help you get started.

"USE YOUR RESOURCES"

TAKE ACTION!

Chapter 10

CONCLUSION

TAKE ACTION

When you file a complaint with the state regarding a nursing home, memory care, or assisted living facility, the state will allow the facilities to develop an action plan to address the issues.

Before filing your complaint, consider whether you are ready to address questions and provide documentation regarding your issue, or if you are reaching out solely based on your emotions.

As you submit your complaint, consider the category that your concern will fall under:

1. Quality of Care
2. Resident Rights
3. Environmental Conditions
4. Staffing Levels
5. Assessment and Care Planning

"What is the deficiency?"
-Isolated Scope
-Pattern Scope
-Widespread Scope

Additionally, consider whether it poses minimal harm or represents an immediate jeopardy.

Long-term care facilities are already familiar with state survey inspections, whether they occur annually or in response to complaints. We know now, they will be given the chance to submit a corrective action plan to address any issues identified. This is why having minutes from resident and family councils is crucial. Any issues raised and documented in the minutes mean that the facility is responsible for addressing your concerns and considering your suggested solutions.

If the facility is developing an action plan for state corrections, where is the documentation demonstrating their efforts to collaborate with the resident and family councils? Keep in mind that the state can review council minutes from the past year.

Collaborate with both staff and management by providing solutions to any concerns. However, always remember the significance of utilizing your family council as a platform to communicate whom you reported your issues to and whether they were resolved. Additionally, this can serve as documentation if others are experiencing similar challenges.

No matter what, make sure to secure a copy of both the original notes and the typed records from resident council and family council meetings. These documents will often be rephrased from what was initially discussed in resident council.

For any inquiries related to this book, please **visit www.youhearmenow.org/contact** and leave a short message.

COMPLAINT

FILING A COMPLAINT WITH
STATE vs FEDERAL GOVERNMENT

The main difference between filing a complaint with the state or federal government for a nursing home is the agency that investigates the complaint and the period of time for a resolution.

State

State survey agencies are usually a part of the States Department of Health and are responsible for investigating complaints about nursing homes. They are required to issue a written decision on the complaint within 60 days unless there are exceptional circumstances. State survey agencies also inspect nursing homes annually and more often if there are complaints or poor performance.

Federal

If the state is not responsive to a complaint, you can file a complaint directly with the regional office of the Centers for Medicare and Medicaid Services (CMS) the agency has 180 days to finish the investigation.

Resources

The Administration on Aging (AoA) within the Department of Health and Human Services (HHS) administers the Long-Term Care Ombudsman Program. The program is mandated by the Older Americans Act to advocate for improvements in long-term care and address complaints.

The Long-Term Care Ombudsman Program; resolve complaints, Educate consumers and long-term care providers about resident rights and good care practices.

Resource Assistance

Resources for long-term care facility assistance, focusing on key state-level support.

1. State Long-Term Care Ombudsman Program

-Free advocates who help residents resolve issues in long-term care facilities.
-Available in every state under federal law.
-Help with complaints, residents' rights, and facility selection.

***This service is for anyone receiving long-term care, memory care, home care, assisted living, and nursing home care.**

2. Medicaid Program

-Each state administers its own Medicaid program.
-Can cover nursing home care and some assisted living costs.
-Contact your state's Medicaid office to learn about eligibility and coverage.

3. State Health Insurance Assistance Program (SHIP)

-Free counseling about Medicare and long-term care insurance options.
-Available in all states.
-Helps navigate coverage and benefits.

4. State Department of Health Elder Affairs

-License and regulate long-term care facilities
-Maintain inspection reports and complaint histories
-Provide facilities ratings and comparison tcols

5. Area Agencies on Aging (AAA)

-Local organizations in every state
-Help connect seniors with long-term care resources
-provide information about facilities and funding option

To find specific resources for your state, you can:

1. Visit eldercare.acl.gov
2. Call 211 for local assistance
3. Contact your state Department of Aging or Elcer Affairs

Book Resources

Nursing Home Secrets Volume One
Research and Insights Gathered From:

Ohio.gov
Aging.ohio.gov
Medicare.gov
Medicaid.gov
CMS.gov
U.S Bureau of Labor Statistics (bls.gov)
Long-Term Care Ombudsman Program
Department of Health & Human Service
The Administration on Aging (AoA)
National Consumer Voice for Quality LTC
National Council on Aging (NCOA)
National Institute on Aging
Personal Experience

If you're feeling overwhelmed and require assistance, I invite you to visit **www.youhearmenow.org/contact** Kindly complete the contact form providing details about the assistance you require.

Special Note

According to the National Council on Aging (NCOA) five million people are affected by elder abuse every single year and the population of adults aged sixty-five and older is expected to increase over the next several decades. This suggests that the issues of elder and nursing home abuse are likely to become even more prominent.

A quote from the National Institute on Aging (NIA):
**"Elder abuse will not stop on its own.
Someone else needs to step in and help."**

Psalm 147:3 (KJV)
"He heals the brokenhearted and binds up their wounds"

www.ingramcontent.com/pod-product-compliance
Lightning Source LLC
LaVergne TN
LVHW022100200926
848481LV00003B/999

* 9 7 9 8 3 4 8 3 2 0 3 8 6 *